The Only Diet

THAT <u>ALWAYS</u> WORKS

Nathaniel Blix

This book is also available in ebook and audiobook versions from online retailers.

Contents

Introduction

The shelves of bookshops groan with diet books. The internet is awash with them. In the light of this, you may think it a bit weird calling this book 'The Only Diet'. It clearly isn't the only diet. Or is it? My excuse for using the phrase is that, really, there *is* only one diet. Those other diet books dress up this basic regime in a whole raft of different ways. But, underneath all the flam and psychobabble, what they all aim for—or should aim for—is the same thing, and that's a healthy diet that's right for you.

What I've tried to do here is to strip the fancy programmes you find in the popular books down to their bare essentials to reveal the basic diet beneath. And I've removed all the prescriptive stuff about what you should eat for lunch and how many baked beans you can have for your dinner. A diet has to work for you, not for some non-existent average citizen. When you follow the Only Diet you can eat whatever you want (as long as you want the right things!)

In the Only Diet, I promise you the most down-to-earth diet book on Earth. It doesn't contain any recipes and has within it only one technical term (you'll find it). The whole thing is based on personal experience, so that's one success story for a start. Also, it's probably the shortest volume on the diet-book shelves. That's slimming in action!

What are my credentials for writing this book? I studied physiology and psychology at university, which gave me the theoretical basics of nutrition. But just as important as this is my experience as a serial dieter. I'll tell you more about this later in the book, but suffice it to say here: I know how difficult it is to lose weight, but I also know how to do it. There's only one way, and this book will tell you what that is.

01. You're fat

You're fat. At any rate, you're fatter than you want to be. In your opinion, you weigh too much. You're too big. Clothes that used to fit you hang in the wardrobe unworn. Every time you open the closet door you think, 'Should I lose a bit of weight so that they will fit me again or should I give up and throw them away?'

You look in a clothes-shop window. You like the way a certain outfit looks on the slim plastic mannequin. You enquire within, ease yourself into a larger version of the same garment and take a look in the mirror. You look terrible. You have the sense not to buy it. Lucky escape!

If that sounds like you, then do yourself a favour. Check yourself on a height-weight chart. These charts are easily available on the internet. Government health departments publish them freely. Measure your height and jump on the scales naked. Check where your height and weight lines intersect on the chart. Coloured bands will tell you roughly where you stand.

You might be classed as 'healthy', 'overweight', 'obese' or perhaps 'very obese'. Of course, you might even be 'underweight'.

If you're 'underweight', this book isn't really for you. Go out and have a great lunch. And then another.

If you're 'healthy', good for you. Carry on what you're doing, but keep this book for when you reach middle age. If you're already there, stop looking so smug.

The rest of you—the rest of *us*, because I too was included in the orange band—if you want to get into the healthy band, keep reading.

02. If you want it, you can have it

Notice how I finished the last chapter: 'if you want to get into the healthy band...'? You might not want to. Some people don't.

Some people are happy being 'overweight'. They think of themselves as a big person, or even a fat person, and they're happy with the way they are. It's unlikely that such a person would have read this book this far. But, if you are, and you did, you can stop reading now. There's nothing here for you. I'm writing for people who are *not* happy with the way they are.

Other people are unhappy being overweight, but they are not prepared to make the effort required to lose it. So they stay fat and get miserable. They may look for easy fixes, such as surgery, drugs, quack medicines, machines that wobble their fat, treatments that sweat the weight off them, all that sort of thing. These treatments are attractive because they offer a gain with no pain (surgery is probably a bit sore). But they are unattractive because they don't work or they're expensive. Anyway, they don't tackle the root of the problem which is an unhealthy lifestyle. After the fat-removing surgery, you'll be back accumulating more for the next surgeon to remove.

That description above—of someone overweight but not prepared to make the effort required to lose it—that was me. But I didn't turn to quack remedies, I just did nothing. This made me even fatter until I decided that enough was enough. I'd actually have to make an effort to get healthy.

There is no gain without pain, not in losing weight, anyway. Isn't it great that those two words rhyme?

To lose weight, you have to want to lose weight. I mean, you have to *really* want to.

I bet you want to live, don't you? You'd be prepared to put quite a lot of effort into staying alive if you found your life threatened in a burning building, for example. Bursting through a door to safety, you'd discover strength you never knew you had. These are the sorts of resources you will need to find if you are to lose weight. Let's not exaggerate, here. I'm not saying that using a couple of extra holes in your belt is as life-threatening as finding your house on fire. What I am saying is that the two situations will require from you—and will get from you—abilities and resources that you don't call upon very often.

If what you're looking for is a magic pill that will take four inches off your waistline while you lie on the beach, then this book isn't for you. If you're not prepared to put in the effort, stop reading now.

I can sense that my readership is dwindling. If you've taken my advice so far, the only people left with me are those who are properly overweight, who want to get healthy and who are prepared to put in some work to make it happen.

If that sounds like you, read on!

03. All about Nat

I am a man, now 62 years old. I'm a reasonably healthy eater. I like vegetables and salad. I don't eat much red meat. I try to avoid salt and fat. However, I love ice cream, cheese, crunchy snacks and alcohol. I love eating and drinking, both socially and for its own sake. I can sit down with friends and eat lunch all Sunday afternoon and I can consume a whole family-sized tub of ice cream alone in front of the television, washing it down with way too many beers or whiskies. Basically, I'm a pig. Oink oink.

Body-wise, I'm probably what they call a mesomorph—not skinny and not inclined to obesity; somewhere in between. Some people just look the skinny type; you can't imagine them putting on weight. Others just look naturally chubby. You wonder if there's a smaller person inside there somewhere, waiting to come out. Often, you conclude that maybe there isn't, they're just built chunky.

I'm not like either of those. I'm tall and in my early adulthood I had a 32-inch waist. On the chart, I was in the healthy band.

Then I started work, as adults tend to do. In my case, most of my jobs have been sedentary. I sat at a desk most of the day. That doesn't mean I didn't walk anywhere. I got the train to my office, so that meant walking to the station at both ends. I walked up the two flights of stairs to my floor instead of taking the elevator.

In my spare time I'd walk quite a bit—in the country, around the city; that sort of thing. I'd mow the lawn, cut the hedge and dig the flower-beds. I'd walk in the park. I led what I considered to be a pretty active urban life.

But, secretly, I was putting on weight. I didn't weigh myself, but I did notice that every few years I was having to shift holes in my belt (I've just realised I've had the same belt for about 15 years!).

The most telling indicator was my tuxedo. I don't know if you have a dinner jacket or other garment with these same characteristics: first, it has a waist-band and second, you don't wear it very often.

I bought my tuxedo when I was about 30. I chose a fairly fashion-free design (without the Osmond lapels) and thought it would last me all my life. I wore it no more than once or twice a year. Every time I went to put it on, I found it was tighter than before. I had the waist-band let out twice before it run out of spare fabric.

What should I do? Buy another tuxedo? No, I decided to lose weight. That was what did it, the tux.

This has happened to me three times in my life. Each time it's the same: my weight creeps up to a point where even I can't deny it. I resolve that I have to do something about it. I go on a diet—the Only Diet—and slim back down to the healthy band.

Then, I have to get my tuxedo trousers taken in. I've had that waistband altered so many times the lady that does it is beginning to complain.

I have embarked on a programme to lose weight three times in my life. The first two times I lost around 12kg (that's 26 pounds), the third time I lost 18kg (40 pounds).

In middle age (When is middle age? I never really know. I'm assuming 45-50ish.) it gets worse because you think, 'My waist is thickening, but so are the waists of all of my friends. It's not good, but it's natural. I'll take the same comments as we all do, but I won't do anything about it.'

This is communal guilt. If all my contemporaries are fat, then it's fine for me to be fat too. Can you see the gap in the argument here? It's quite big. You got it—it's your body we're talking about here, not your friends'. Can you find any comfort in being able to say, in later life, 'I was unattractive and found it difficult to climb a flight of stairs without stopping half-way for a breather, but at least it was the same for my friends.'?

I don't think so.

Anyway, getting back to me, if my weight goes up and down like a yo-yo, my diet—the Only Diet—can't be any good, is that what you're thinking? It's a good challenge. My response to it is this: if I'd stuck to the diet after losing so much weight the first and second times, I could have controlled my weight at a healthy level. But I didn't. I got back into bingeing on ice cream and beer, cheese and wine and all the rest.

This time it's different. This time, after I lost the 18kg, I have stayed on the diet and my weight has not wavered from the healthy band. I've taken my own advice and established the Only Diet not as a one-off programme of quick weight loss, but a rest-of-my-lifetime approach to healthy eating. Losing weight is just too difficult. I don't want to have to do it again, so I'm keeping an eye on the dial and not letting the needle swing into the danger zone.

Never again. I've promised myself.

04. The voices

This chapter is as close as I'll get to psychobabble in this book. It's not based on any accepted psychological law or theory. It has no scientific basis and there's no evidence to support it, so far as I know.

Where did it come from? I made it up.

That's being a bit flip. Let me try to explain more clearly. 'The voices' come from my experience. When I lose weight, the following is what it seems like to me:

Food is great; drinks are delicious. They're designed that way. Prepared foods are formulated to be tasty; they're intended to make you want to eat them. Recipes are designed to result in palatable dishes. It's all so obvious. Eating is one of life's pleasures. We do it with friends. We pay money to do it in restaurants, sometimes ridiculous amounts of money. Eating is friends, family, culture, life.

Exercise is hard work. When you walk from the bus stop to the shop, you take the shortest route. When you need a new light-bulb, you don't walk to the corner-store, you take the car. You stand on the escalator. Why would you take the stairs if there's an elevator? OK, you want to save time, but also you're lazy. You like things that save you effort. You don't cut the grass with shears, you use an electric mower. Think of how many electric motors you have in your house. I even have an electrical machine to juice a lemon. It saves me twisting my hand a few times on a glass lemon squeezer. We have little motors to wind our car windows up and down, because we're too lazy to turn a crank handle. It's ridiculous.

You know all this.

You also know that eating too much food makes you fat. And you know that exercise is good for you.

There's an inconsistency here. We 'know' things that are contradictory. Our brains carry two sets of conflicting urges.

Food is good, exercise is hard. Exercise is good, food is dangerous.

The way this seems to me is that I have two voices in my head, each of which presents to 'me' one of these two conflicting arguments.

They're not really voices. I don't actually hear them talking to me. I don't need to be locked up quite yet. Calling them 'voices' is just a convenient way of expressing their separate and contradictory messages, and their persuasiveness. Really, they're 'ways of thinking'.

One voice tells me: 'Order the super-size burger, go for seconds, eat the cheese, drink the beer. They taste good. You deserve it. You're not fat. You can always diet tomorrow. You never liked that suit that no longer fits. You have to take a taxi because you're late. You can't run in those shoes. You're not the sporty type. The gym's too embarrassing and expensive. You're not a natural athlete. You're no fatter than most of your friends. It's natural to fill out at your age. Eating and drinking are social past-times; they're what hold communities together. Have fun; it's what life's all about.'

The other voice tells me: 'Go easy on the french fries. You only need a small helping of dessert to get the experience. Limit yourself to two beers a day. Cut the fat off that steak. Leave the chicken skin. You're looking pudgy in the face. You're beginning to hang over the belt of your jeans. You won't fit an aeroplane seat soon. You think that's attractive to the opposite sex? It's not healthy; think of the extra work your heart has to do. What kind of example is that to your kids? Can you still knock a ball around with them? Lose some weight, get into shape. Do whatever it takes to get back to the healthy band and stay there.'

Any of this sound familiar? If not, then my advice is to 'listen' out for these voices. You won't actually hear anything, but trying to hear them may help you resolve the confused mash of urges swilling around inside your head into two opposing arguments. Try it. Listen for the arguments on one side and the other. I found that helpful. Ultimately, it's essential to identify your enemy before you attempt to overthrow him. You see what I mean?

Let's call these opposing camps the 'good voice' and the 'bad voice'. It won't come as much of a surprise to you that we want the arguments of the good voice to prevail over those of the bad voice. If that's a fight you think is just not worth the effort, then stop reading now.

If you're with me in wanting to defeat that naughty old bad voice, no matter what it takes, then read on.

05. The way we were

It's worth remembering not only who we are but who we were. Thinking back through evolution can often provide us with insights into why we act the way we do. I'm not taking you back to amoebas or worms, or even as far into the past as when our ancestors were fish or apes. A few hundreds of thousands of years will do, to when we were human-shaped hunter-gatherers. In those days we didn't farm, we hunted and, er, gathered.

It's tough being a hunter. The tasty animals you want to catch would prefer not to be caught. And it's no picnic being a gatherer, either. The birds get up pretty early and take the best berries, the pigs dig out the juiciest roots before you get there. Then, without warning, the rain doesn't come for a month and there's no salad to be found for miles. It's a wonder our ancestors didn't just give up and go home.

A hunter-gatherer is lucky if he can hunt and gather enough to keep his family alive. There's no excess, no gluttony, no danger of junior back in the cave getting fat.

It's pretty certain that, of the two voices I discussed in the previous chapter, the bad voice is the older one, the one we evolved first. This is the only voice that a hunter-gatherer would have needed. In those days we would have called it something like a 'survival' voice rather than bad, and it was probably saying slightly different things in those days, but there's no mistaking it as the ancestor of the bad voice we hear today.

In a hunter-gatherer's head, the survival voice would be saying things like: 'Eat while you have the chance, there may be no food tomorrow. Eat the fat, it will give you energy for your next hunt. Look for sweet things because sugar is a good source of energy and sweet fruits get gobbled up fast by others. Don't let the next guy get the berries; keep them for yourself and your family. Eat salt if you find it because it's essential and hard to come by.'

There was no 'good' voice because none was needed. Hunter-gatherers didn't consider the argument 'Just one more spoonful of ice cream won't do you any harm' worth bothering with because they didn't have ice cream or anything like it.

The 'survival' voice was very useful to our hunter-gather ancestors. It told them to make the most of their opportunities and conserve energy. It helped them survive.

As we found ways, through agriculture and other technologies, of harnessing nature to produce huge food surpluses, so the survival voice became superfluous. We didn't need it any longer, but it was still there. It became a bad voice. We found that we needed to call up a good voice to temper the excesses that the new bounty made possible.

For completeness, it's worth reminding ourselves that the conditions I've described here are the ones to be found in the industrialised (rich) nations. In many others, food is still scarce for many people. I'm glad to have cleared that up.

In conclusion, think of your good voice as the modern, civilised, wealthy argument against a much more ancient urge, one that we needed to survive when times were bad, but which is no longer appropriate. Before, the way to stay alive was to eat everything that came our way, especially energy-rich foods containing fat and sugar. Now that we have these things in plenty, everything is reversed and the way to stay healthy is to resist much of the temptation with which we are presented.

06. What is food, anyway?

Why do we enjoy eating? Our bodies have evolved this idea that it's good to eat because, basically, we need to eat. If it wasn't enjoyable, we might not bother, then where would we be?

But why do we *need* to eat? Any ideas? It's pretty simple. The answer is that food gives us two essential things.

First, it gives us materials. Our bodies are made of chemicals, some of which don't last forever, so if we're growing, we need more of them and, even if we're not, we need replacements. These chemicals are either structural—those which make up the fabric of our bodies, like bone, skin, muscle and so on; or process—those which take part in chemical reactions, like enzymes, hormones and such like.

The body is remarkably good at processing chemicals. We can make quite a lot of the ones we need from the ones that come to us in food. For example, we can make human proteins from all the non-human proteins we get from eating chickens, pigs, beans and so on. We can make fat from carbohydrate, and vice versa. It's very clever.

But there are some things we can't make. Minerals and some vitamins are beyond our alchemy, so we have to make sure that these are present in our diet.

To get all the chemicals we need, our bodies thrive when our diet is as varied as possible. If you specialise too much in a small number of foods, then your body may find itself short of the ingredients it needs to make the right chemicals. So here's a big lesson: a healthy diet is a varied diet. Eat as many different things as you can. I call this diet diversity. (Actually, I don't, but I thought it might make a good sound-bite.)

How koalas survive solely on eucalyptus leaves I have no idea. They must have evolved super-ingenious ways of making koala protein out of gum-tree protein. Don't try this at home.

Remember I said we needed food for two reasons? That was the first. The second is because it gives us energy.

Moving, being warm, being alive at all—these all need energy. In a motor car, energy is the difference between the metal, plastic and glass construction that comes off the factory production line and the F1 machine as it hurtles past the chequered flag.

When you're a hunter-gatherer, energy is your most precious commodity. Don't waste it. Don't run if you can walk; don't stand if you can sit. Conserve your energy. And look for foods that contain the most energy—seeds, roots and meat. When you find them, eat all you can. In the summer, take advantage of seasonal foods; they won't be around in the winter.

Energy was so important to our ancestors that our bodies were designed not to waste it. And we still have the same bodies. If you eat more than necessary for your immediate usage, your body will never ever discard it; it will store it away for when times are hard. It does this in a number of ways, but the one that's important to us right now is by making fat.

So what foods are good for us and which foods are bad?

Excuse me, but this reminds me of when I was a science schoolteacher and my pupils would ask me questions like, 'What's the point of a mosquito?' The answer to a question like that is that it's the wrong question.

Any nutritious food might be good for you if eaten as part of a varied diet, yet not so good if it was all you ate. Any food laded with the classic no-nos is going to be bad for you if you eat it all the time, but consumed occasionally it's not really going to be a problem.

It's a lot more meaningful to talk about good and bad diets than good or bad foods. Any reasonable food is fine—even the ones people tell you are bad for you—as long as it's part of a varied diet. It's diet diversity that's important. Oops, I used that catch-phrase again!

Oh, and the answer to the question about the mosquito is: ask the mosquito. Or if you're feeling poetic: it's part of life's rich tapestry.

07. Something's burning

In the previous chapter, we discovered the importance of energy. How do our bodies obtain energy? Pretty much as you would expect, they do it by burning things they get from food.

'Burning' sounds as if it may involve a fire. But the way our bodies do it (and the bodies of practically all other living things, incidentally) is by conducting the process in a very controlled way, to maximise the usable energy that comes out of it, while minimising the heat it generates and so avoiding a flame. The process is called 'respiration' and that could be the first and last 'technical' term you'll find in this book.

Respiration does make some heat, as you'll know if you've ever speeded up the respiration in your own body by running for a bus.

What is it that we burn? Cars burn gasoline; stoves burn wood; bodies burn glucose. It's as simple as that. Glucose is our fuel. We get glucose from our food. You don't actually have to eat spoonfuls of the sweet white powder. Luckily, our bodies can make glucose from any of the major food categories.

We use lots of different units to measure energy. The useful one for dieters is the calorie. Technically, it should be written with a capital C to show that it's really a thousand times bigger than a real calorie, but most people don't bother, so I won't either. A big-C calorie is sometimes called a kilocalorie, or kcal, meaning a thousand calories. But let's press on.

We need different amounts of energy at different times and clearly it would be inconvenient if we had to adjust our food intake accordingly (imagine having to eat a bread roll before being able to run for the bus, for example). So, like an off-road car in the desert with its gas tank inside and reserve can strapped on the back, we hold reserves of fuel for immediate, medium-term and long-term storage.

The one that's important here is our long-term store. To store energy for the future, our bodies use fat. You have to admire our bodies' genius because fat is very efficient for this purpose. You know what fat looks like. It's the hard, juicy, white stuff on the edge of a steak. Your fat looks exactly like that. Of course, fat has to be put somewhere. You can see as well as I can where it goes—actually quite a few places, but most obviously under the skin.

There's a two-way relationship between the glucose in our blood and the fat beneath our skin. If we take in more food than we need, this will increase the glucose in our blood. Since it isn't required just yet, our bodies convert it to fat and store it away around our waistlines for later, straining our new trousers. If we use up more than we take in, our bodies convert some fat to glucose, which is then respired. This eases the pressure on our belts and causes our trousers to fall down.

That last bit was a joke, but when I lost 18kg a couple of years ago, my waistline shrank from 38 to 34 inches, and actually my trousers did occasionally require extra support.

Pause for amusing image of Nat.

08. Clearing out the store

We've already established that you're fatter than you feel you should be, because I told you back in Chapter 1 to stop reading if you're not. How did you get that way? Well, I don't know you, but I do know how you got to be fat. It was because you ate too much for the amount of energy you were using. Sorry, but it's true.

Different people need different amounts of energy, according to how active they are. An ice-hockey player or sugar-cane harvester wouldn't last long on a diet that was just right for a desk-bound accountant. My guess is that you got it the other way around. You're the equivalent of a desk-bound accountant and you were on an ice-hockey diet. I know I was.

'Whoopee!' said your body (not really, but stay with the argument for a while). 'Whoopee! Lots of lovely food, containing lots of precious energy. I'm going to store that for when it's needed. Hang on while I convert most of it to fat and tuck it away under the skin, with all the rest.' That's what your body said.

The trouble is, it wasn't ever needed. You're still a desk-bound accountant with no plans to play ice-hockey or harvest sugar-cane any time soon. So the energy is still there, around your middle, stored for a rainy day that never came.

So what are you going to do about it? You've got a lot of energy stored up that you don't need. It's pretty obvious, but I'll spell it out anyway. There are two things to be done.

First, you have to eat less. Consider this:

There are three amounts of food you can regularly eat. You can eat:

More than you need, in which case you will put on weight.

The amount you need, in which case your weight will be stable.

Less than you need, in which case you will lose weight.

Second, you have to exercise more. If you're still with me, consider this:

Exercise will increase the amount of energy you need, and will make the first action—eating less—much less painful.

So there you have it. It's simple. To lose weight you must eat less and exercise more. You must do both of these until the amount of energy you're using is greater than the amount you're eating.

'Piffpaff and fiddlesticks,' I hear you cry. 'Is that the Only Diet? I could've worked that one out for myself!'

Well, actually, yes, that is the only diet and you could have worked it out for yourself, but you didn't. So stop complaining and read on.

By the way, before you do: I've made a number of references to fat being stored around the waist. It is stored there, but it goes to a lot of other places too—legs, backside and so on. When you lose weight, you will be surprised to find that you lose it from practically everywhere. I had to get my wedding ring made smaller because my finger slimmed down so much.

You want to do that?

OK, you can go to the next chapter now.

09. Don't even think about dessert

That's what it feels like sometimes when you're trying to lose weight. It feels as if all food is evil and you're not allowed to touch it. Certainly, stopping eating altogether would get you to your ideal weight quickest, but it's not a good idea. It wouldn't be possible for anyone but a monk and anyway food is still there to be enjoyed.

Your objective at this stage should be to establish a new way of eating. Say to yourself: 'Whatever I was doing before was no good. It didn't work because it made me fatter than I want. If I'm going to get back to the healthy band (and I'm completely determined to do this), I'm going to have to change. The status quo is not an option. However, I still enjoy the taste of food and its role as a social enabler. So what does my future diet look like?'

Well you tell me. The Only Diet isn't one of those books that tells you to have two prawns for lunch and some lightly poached salmon for dinner. You may hate fish. You may be a vegetarian. The Only Diet is the one that's right for you, and only you know what you will be able to stick to. However, here are some principles:

Stay away from fatty foods

Cut down on carbohydrates, especially sugar

Choose white or pink before red meat

Banish the salt cellar

Tuck into green vegetables

Eat fruit

Drink lots of water

Increase your diet diversity

Take a multivitamin/mineral pill

As well as the little rules above, there's also the big overriding rule: eat less. We know you were eating too much, because it made you fat. Sorry, but you have to get into the habit of eating less.

10. Raise your glasses

A word about alcoholic drinks: I'm not going to deal here about the effects of the alcohol itself; there are plenty of other sources for that kind of information. But alcoholic drinks also contain energy so should concern anyone who's trying to lose weight.

A tot of whisky has about the same calories as a rasher of bacon; a glass of wine is about as calorific as a sausage. A small beer is somewhere in between. You drink four pints of beer, that's half a dozen sausages.

The thing about drinks is that they deliver calories but don't make you feel full. So you can take in all the energy you need from a hearty meal and still have room for quite a few drinks. That's 'extra' calories that'll make you put on weight. Alcohol will make your efforts to lose weight more difficult. If you can't live without a gin and tonic after work, OK, life is for living, but ration yourself to a sensible amount and choose calorie-free mixers.

I love drink and consume far too much of it. To lose weight, the rule I adopt is: only two small beers a day unless we go out or have friends over.

This actually taught me that I don't need as much alcohol as I thought I did. These days, I quite often go without. Well, occasionally.

I give up drink entirely in February. I chose this month because it's the shortest, yet I can still tell people that I gave up for a month.

The important thing for weight loss is that you have to include your drink consumption in your daily calorie quota. Sorry, but life's tough.

I discovered that one of the pleasures of drinking is the ceremony and having something to do while I'm talking or watching a movie. Sometimes these days I satisfy these desires by drinking plain soda water. I put it in a fine cut-glass tumbler with lots of ice, drop in some lime juice or maybe some Angostura bitters and pretend that I'm having a real drink. It sometimes works, it sometimes doesn't and I top up with gin. When it does work, I've saved calories.

Cutting down on drink also saves you money. If that's not important to you, then try trading up instead. Order a glass of expensive wine instead of a bottle of plonk. Or go for one measure of super-deluxe single malt instead of three standard Scotches. It'll make you feel swanky and save you some precious calories.

11. Midnight feast, anyone?

I'm sure you've heard lots of people telling you that if you want to lose weight you should eat a hearty breakfast and toy with a lettuce leaf for your evening meal. The argument is that you burn food faster during the day, so it isn't laid down as fat.

I suspect that this is yet another example of wanting something for nothing: 'You don't have to eat less to lose weight; you just have to shift your consumption around the clock.'

Maybe it works and maybe it doesn't. If it does, my guess is that the effect is very small. In my experience, the important thing is the total amount of energy in your food, not the time of day you eat it.

I have tried the big breakfast approach, but I found it just made me hungrier at lunchtime and ravenous in the evening, so I quickly gave up.

The approach I take is to have nothing for breakfast, to limit my lunch to 500 calories and my dinner to 1,000 calories because that is what suits my lifestyle.

The chances are you're different. You may be an early riser and have time to kill before you start the business of the day, in which case a big breakfast may suit you fine. Or it may be that lunch is the important occasion for you or, like me, dinner. Whatever. Fit your eating pattern in with the rest of your life; you're supposed to be establishing a *sustainable* new healthy lifestyle here, one that works for you. How can you make your lifestyle healthy, that's the question, not how can I change to an ideal regime that might suit some diet-freak who doesn't really exist.

Although it's undoubtedly the total number of calories you eat that's important, it will help you keep track of your intake if you limit your eating to regular mealtimes. I used to be a terrible grazer. I'd eat chocolate, ice cream, crisps and practically any kind of packaged snack all the time. Then I'd go ahead and have my regular meals on top. Try reading the calorie content on the back of a packet of potato crisps. It's a lot, and you have to factor it in to your daily quota. How would you rather take your calories, in a fatty, salt-laden snack or as a pile of crunchy vegetables? Yes, OK, I know you probably opted for the potato chips, but that's not going to get you where you want to go, is it? Mend your ways and read on!

12. It's a gas

One of the most important insights you will get from this book is the answer to this simple question: when you lose weight, where does it go?

It's common sense that something must leave your body to make it lighter. But what is it and how does it leave?

Most people will tell you that you must lose weight through your pee or poo. (I hope you don't mind if I use children's names for these vital bodily functions; they're probably preferable in this context to the medical or scatological equivalents.) But actually you don't. A person losing weight does no more poo than a person gaining it. Pee (and water balance generally) is a more complicated issue, but for the purposes of this insight, we can safely ignore it.

The truth is that we breathe the weight out.

That fat I talked about in earlier chapters, that's what has to go. We break it down into glucose and then respire it. Like all organic 'burning' processes, respiring glucose produces carbon dioxide which we breathe out as a gas.

You're shocked. You're asking, 'How can I lose weight by breathing out such a light thing as a gas? It'll take centuries.'

Not true. Carbon dioxide isn't light. Actually, it's quite heavy, as you'll know if you've ever lifted a block of dry ice, which of course is solid carbon dioxide. As a gas, it still weighs the same, it just takes up more space.

Since we lose weight by breathing out carbon dioxide, it follows that the more we breathe out, the more weight we lose. Do you see where this is going? What makes us breathe more heavily—both deeper and faster? You got it, exercise! That's what the next chapter is all about.

By the way, don't get the idea that hyperventilating while lying on a sun-lounger is going to make you lose weight. Respiration drives breathing, not the other way around. Getting puffed at rest will only make you black out. Don't say I didn't warn you.

13. On your bike

You don't exercise enough.

I'm talking about you.

If you did exercise enough, you wouldn't be fat. The thing about exercise is that it uses up energy and establishes you at a higher level of energy need. This means you can get away with reducing your food intake less.

It's also good for you. You're not made of muscle so you can flop in front of the television, employing only the little muscles in your thumb to operate the remote control. You're meant to use your muscles to move around. If you don't use them, your body will wonder why it's bothering to maintain them. It will start breaking them down for something useful, like boosting your fat store, and we don't want that, do we?

No, we don't.

All exercise is the same, but my advice would be to:

Slowly increase the amount you do to a level that challenges you.

Do something measurable.

Do it regularly.

This last time, when I lost the 18kg, I joined a gym. I've never liked gyms. I'm self-conscious in front of all the rippling muscles and I find the machines boring to work on. I've forced myself to get over all of that. Now it's a routine that I go through. Me, I go to the gym five days a week for about 80 minutes each time. I'm retired. I can afford the time. You have a busy life. There's no way you could fit that in, that's what you're thinking.

Well, what could you fit in? How important is this to you? Surely there's some slack in your schedule somewhere, or some activity you currently find time for which is less important than your health? I'll leave it with you. But get into a routine. If it's three times a week, make those three sessions appointments in your diary that can't be broken by pesky business meetings or dates with your friends. Work around your commitment to yourself.

Here's what I do. When I go to the gym, I use three exercise machines and eight weight machines. First I do time on a bike, then four weight exercises, then I pull on a rowing machine, followed by the last four weight exercises. Finally, I walk on the treadmill. I always do exactly the same amount of work on each machine: the same calories on the machines; the same weights and the same repetitions on the lifting exercises. That way I can't cheat. If I stopped short I would feel I'd cheated myself. I'd feel the bad voice had won a round against the good voice and that, as we now know, would be completely unacceptable.

It's boring and time-consuming, so I use the time to think. If I have a problem that needs thinking through, I put it off until I go to the gym the next morning. There I am on the bike, sorting out my insurance policies, investments, ideas for books, family issues, whatever. That's how I get over the boredom. I forget what my legs are doing and concentrate on something completely disconnected. I must look weird, and so will you, but this is important so get over it.

You don't have to do this. You don't have to go to a gym. But you do have to exercise. This might be playing a sport of some kind, running round the streets, looking athletic in the park, challenging yourself to some physical achievement, in a team or alone, anything; anything, really that gets your body moving. Team sports are good because you have to turn up otherwise you let your team mates down. It's a good way of overcoming discouraging messages from the bad voice.

Remember your objective: do something that makes you puffed, and do it so regularly that your bad voice can't knock you off schedule.

While you're huffing and puffing in your chosen exercise tell yourself this: 'With every breath I take I'm losing weight.' Feel the heavy carbon dioxide leaving your body and changing the climate. Ha ha.

Turn up the speed or the effort and you breathe faster. That's because you have more carbon dioxide to get rid of, and we all know how heavy that stuff is.

14. Measure and manage

Any person in business will tell you that if you don't measure it, you can't manage it. They're talking about things like costs and risks, but the same holds true for diets. Get into the numbers.

First, food. Acquaint yourself with the calories in the foods you eat. I'm not going to give you a chart of the figures because they're easily obtainable in books or on the internet. Read the nutrition content labels on prepared foods. Pretty soon you'll be able to make a reasonably good estimate of the energy content of any dish of food.

Decide on your target total calorie intake for the day. Again, there are charts for this, but you need a figure that's right for you. I'm a big man who works out six days a week and I know that if I stop at 1,500 calories a day, I will lose weight at a rate of about 100g a day (that's about a pound every five days). By trial and error, you will find a figure that's right for you. To make it easy, start at 1,000 or 1,500 or maybe 2,000 calories a day, according to your sex and size, and work up or down until you're losing weight at about the same rate as me.

Having a daily total, and knowing the values of different foods, will help you make judgements about what you eat. Is it worth eating that chocolate cake/lamb chop when I could have a huge helping of my favourite salad instead? Or whatever. Juggle around with the things you eat to stay within the same limit, not forgetting the basic rules set out in Chapter 9.

Second, exercise. The value of measuring your exercise is so that you can equate it to the amount you're eating. But it will also make it more difficult for your bad voice to persuade you to cheat. If you work out in a gym, ignore the time clock on your machine and concentrate on the calorie counter. Time doesn't matter; it's energy that counts. On my three exercise machines, I clock up 1,000 calories a day altogether. If I'm only eating 1,500 a day, it's easy to see that I don't have to do much more for the rest of the day before I start losing weight.

A gramme of fat can store about nine calories, so those 1,000 calories I do every day in the gym burn about 100g of fat. In the old units, a pound of body fat can store 3,500 calories, so if I pedal 500 calories a day, I'll lose a pound a week.

If your exercise routine is in the park or on the tennis court or football pitch (or whatever), use the internet to find out how many calories someone of your weight is using per hour.

Third, you. An essential part of the Only Diet is to keep close track of your success. You will need some scales on which to weigh yourself, a piece of paper and a pen. On the paper, draw a grid with two columns. In the first, write the date on each row, a day at a time. In the second, record your weight. Yes, you're going to weigh yourself every day and you're going to write it down.

Weigh yourself at the same time every day. The best time is when you get up. (I was going to say 'in the morning' but, heck, you could be working the night shift.) Go to the toilet first, so you're sure it's you that you're measuring, take off all your clothes and step on to the scales. Gasp in amazement at how much you've lost. You actually lose quite a lot overnight from just breathing and water balancing.

If you're a whizz with Excel, you can punch your daily weight into a spreadsheeet and draw a graph. This will show you immediately if it's all going according to plan or if you're slacking off.

Decide on a target weight and write this on your chart. Get the target weight from one of the height-weight charts discussed in Chapter 1. Choose a target that's realistic for you and preferably go for one that gets you into the healthy band.

If you're very fat, this may be a long shot and you may decide that coming down a couple of bands is achievement enough. You have to decide this for yourself, but everyone's long-term goal, if this is worth doing at all, should be to get into the healthy height-weight ratio band.

A refinement of the chart idea is to map out your progress in advance from your start, today, to your target, say a few months off. This will need perhaps four columns—one for the date, one for your target weight each day (decreasing by, say, 100g a day), the third for your actual weight recorded each day and the last for your reward (or punishment)—that's a tick or a cross according to whether you're on track or slipping behind.

Monitoring your food intake, exercise and body weight like this will give you a real feel for how your body works. You'll find that, after a night out drinking (we're still human), you weigh much less the next day than you thought you would. That's because alcohol dries you out. The following day, after you've replaced all the water you lost, annoyingly you'll be back up. You'll discover the effects of being constipated for a couple of days; also of when this condition eases. You'll be surprised how much weight you lose on a long walk in the country.

Once you're in tune with the relationships between food, exercise and body weight, you'll find it a lot easier to control your diet and get the result you're looking for.

15. The pangs!

It's easy to write this stuff about the Only Diet, but not so easy to follow its advice. Believe me, I know; I've done it and I'm still doing it every day.

For me, the worst thing is the hunger. After the first few days on a lot less food than I've been used to, the bad voice is screaming in my head, 'Give up now! Walk away! No-one will know. What have you got to lose?' I feel hungry nearly all day. I feel hungry after a meal. I fall asleep at night feeling hungry.

Under the circumstances the only crumbs of comfort my good voice can offer are these two points: first, when your body is used to enjoying a certain amount of food every day for many years, it's not surprising that it reacts by feeling hungry when that amount is sharply reduced. The feeling will ease as your new regime becomes established. Second, my good voice reasons that I've enjoyed years of over-indulgence; I've had the party and now is the time to pay the bill. Gee, thanks, good voice.

Did you find that comforting? It was all I had. Maybe your good voice can find more convincing arguments to help you with the pangs of hunger.

If not, there are some practical things you can do about hunger. The idea is to fool your body into thinking it has been fed without actually introducing much more in the way of calories. I look for bulky foods that will fill me up without pushing me over my daily energy limit.

Cucumbers are quite good. Don't slice them; just gnaw them like an apple. I also binge on celery and iceberg lettuce. Raw carrot's good too. It's good to get some variety.

I hope this isn't sounding too much like other diets. I promised not to give you recipes or tell you what to eat. Whatever, you may have a better idea about what bulky, non-calorific foods are best for staving off your hunger pains.

One major breakthrough in diet technology that I'm quite proud of is the use of fizzy drinks, or sodas as they call them in some places. I'm referring to the zero-calorie versions of your favourite carbonated beverages.

When I feel so hungry I could eat the carpet, I stave off my desire by drinking a glass or two of no-calorie soda and find that the sweetness and the bulk of all that gas seems to fool my body into thinking it's full. When I first hit upon this ruse, I used to drink cola but found that this contained so much caffeine I couldn't sleep at night.

So I switched to ginger beer.

I was in London at the time and I'm thinking that ginger beer may be an exclusively British beverage, which is a shame because it worked like magic. Also, it tastes great. No caffeine, no calories and it made me feel full. It became so important to my weight loss, I nearly called this programme the Ginger Beer Diet.

Let's not get down-hearted. In countries where you can't get ginger beer, I have no doubt that other calorie-free fizzy drinks are available that would work just as well. But look out for the caffeine.

16. Never give up

The Only Diet is for life. It should become your new way of thinking about food, both when you're on your way to your target weight and the healthy band, and afterwards.

When you reach your target weight, you can slacken off a little on the starvation rations, but don't give up the basic principles of healthy eating, diet diversity, exercise and careful monitoring of not only your energy input and output but also your weight. Let these become habits. Weigh yourself every morning for the rest of your life.

Take it from me, for years your 'natural' way of life has been to eat too much. When you reach your lower target weight you could easily revert to this behaviour unless you keep up the monitoring. Even if you manage to overcome your bad voice, it will still be there, silenced perhaps for months, but still ready to spring back into action as soon as your good voice relaxes.

Be vigilant, maintain the habit, keep the bad voice at bay, never give up.

17. How was it for you?

Did the Only Diet work for you? How much weight did you lose? Do you feel better? Was it tough? (probable answer: yes) Are you keeping it up? Is it a habit for life? Have you regressed?

Don't forget: this is the Only Diet That Always Works. If you're not losing weight, you must have slipped up somewhere. Go back to Chapter 1 and start again.

Meanwhile, it would be great to keep in touch. Please become my friend on Facebook and share your weight-loss and healthy-eating successes with others!

facebook.com/profile.php?id=100002583867054

If you want a personal response, write to me:

nat.blix@hotmail.com